What God says about Abortion

Understanding Abortion using Biblical Studies and Christian Scriptures on human life, Forgiveness, Consequences and Way Forward

Gedaliah Shay

© Copyright 2020- Alpha Zuriel Publishing All rights reserved

The content contained within this book may not be reproduced, duplicated or transmitted without direct written permission from the author or the publisher.

Under no circumstances will any blame or legal responsibility be held against the publisher, or author, for any damages, reparation, or monetary loss due to the information contained within this book; either directly or indirectly.

Scripture taken from the New King James Version®. Copyright © 1982 by Thomas Nelson. Used by permission. All rights reserved.

Legal Notice:

This book is copyright protected. This book is only for personal use. You cannot amend, distribute, sell, use, quote or paraphrase any part, or the content within this book, without the consent of the author or publisher.

Table of Contents

Introduction 1

Chapter One 5

Chapter Two 26

Chapter Three 51

Chapter Four 70

Chapter Five 84

Conclusion 92

Prayer 101

Introduction

What does the bible really teach about abortion?"

As Christians, our faith is based on the understanding that human life is precious and valuable to God. It is the sole reason why he sent his son, Jesus Christ to save us from eternal damnation and suffering.

The bible scriptures hold truths that are proof of God's love for mankind. Having made man in his image and likeness, all humans representatives of the glory of God. This affirms the unique value of all human life.

This book is built upon the premise of the sixth commandment—**"You** shall not murder" (Ex. 20:13)—and condemns every form of destruction or termination of a human life at any stage of its development from the point of conception to the point of death.

Hence, this book stands strongly against abortion, and affirms that it is an allowable option only when the life of the mother-to-be is genuinely threatened by the continuation of the pregnancy. Christians are mobilized worldwide to speak against this atrocity of abortion and push that the legislation in regards to abortion reflects the truth of scripture and places value on human life.

Abortion is one very controversial topic worldwide, and different people stand for and against it, with their own reasons.

This book doesn't in anyway seek to condemn those who have been involved in abortions, but the action and dissuade people from engaging in it by teaching the possible dangers.

The scripture is very clear on the fact that murder is forbidden by God. Every life is a gift and should be cherished as such. Murder is not only the devaluation of human life but waste of God's precious gift. It is a grave sin that is highly consequential and punishable by God. This book teaches these consequences explicitly.

As a Christian, I am of the belief that there is no excuse that is worth taking a human life and exposing oneself to the terrible consequences. Believers should also show compassion and not condemnation to those who have had abortions. Scripture points us to love and not castigate.

This and many more truths we will be looking at in a more elaborate light as we try to find out, "What God says about abortion."

As you go through the pages of this book, I pray that you may find light and truth!

Chapter One

Scriptural Definition of Abortion

71% of young unmarried girls in the U.S have had an abortion at least once in their life. It is the new normal in society. Just as simple as it is to hear people say they go to treat themselves in the hospital. People do it without a second thought and try to feel normal. Once a lady finds out that she's pregnant, she just walks into the nearest hospital and evacuates the fetus from her womb, like a person would remove a brain tumor!

Many activists have risen to fight this act and make people understand how wrong it is while facing direct contention with the top proponents. These proponents are very violent and pigheaded about their views on abortion.

Several years ago, abortion was one concept that people never really talked about. It wasn't popular, and there were unconventional ways of terminating unwanted pregnancies as far back as the 1800's.

Some of these methods include the use of abortifacient herbs, applying abdominal pressure, and the use of sharp instruments, amongst others. These practices were quite painful and dangerous, and only a few persons were willing to submit themselves to the pain just to get rid of their unwanted fetus.

Eventually, when technology began to influence the world system, and more conventional and less painful methods of abortion were developed, many persons threw it to the wind and began to champion the cause. Abortion laws started to arise in different countries, but that didn't stop the practice from thriving, even in secret. Some doctors opened secret health centers where they helped determined women terminate their pregnancy. In developing countries, where abortion laws only strive on paper, we have persons walking in and out of hospitals every day of the week to have abortions. In a year, over a thousand abortions are done, which the government knows nothing about.

At some point, the proponents of abortion began to gain recognition as they came out with the campaign for women's rights recognition. As usual, the majority rule won, and in a few years, the once terrible practice was legalized, and people were free to practice and carry on the act publicly.

The abortion rate has started to drop over the years as there are now contraceptives that people use to prevent pregnancy and family planning technology solutions. These technology systems have replaced the abortion system. However, mistakes still happen as contraceptives are not 100% guaranteed. This mistake as it is usually called, is eliminated by abortion.

Why People Commit Abortion

The decision to have abortion is a very complex and sensitive one. It is not as likely as many people think it to be. There are several reasons why people commit abortion. People always have reasons to carry out this act, no matter the number of times they do it. Below is listed a few reasons why women commit abortion. We are not going to validate or attack any of the reasons. We will just highlight and explain them to grant us a clear picture and help us understand popular reasons why women terminate their pregnancy prematurely.

Understanding why women have abortion will help us know how well to address the concept fully from that light, using the scriptures

- **Bad timing, not prepared.** This is one of the most popular reasons people give for aborting their baby. Associated reasons could be that the pregnancy interferes with their educational or career goals. We have many career women who are present have had to eliminate many mistake pregnancies.
- **Not emotionally and mentally prepared**: This set

of people give the excuse that they are not ready for the responsibility of motherhood

- **Rape case:** 98% of pregnant rape victims abort their baby because of the pain and trauma.
- **Partner related reasons:** In situations when a lady gets pregnant in an abusive or new relationship, she hurriedly gets rid of the baby. She is scared of having a child for someone who might turn them and the baby down and eventually walk away, leaving her a single mother.
- **Health related issues**: There are cases when the

health of the mother and fetus is poor. Most times, abortion is prescribed by the doctor. Such form of abortion is fully endorsed worldwide.

Abortion involves the termination of a growing fetus from a woman. WHO, the national center for Health, and the Centers for Disease Control and prevention define abortion as the termination of pregnancy before 20 weeks of gestation. At 20 weeks of gestation, the baby is already growing, and that seed is a child already. Terminating that seed is preventing the growth of a child. However, the pro-life activists claim that taking contraceptives immediately after conception is abortion and termination of a human life.

This definition has caused a solid uproar in the western world.

Meanwhile, Abortion-right movements in seeking to justify their movement chant that the bible says nothing about abortion. They lay their claim that in all book of the bible, abortion is not mentioned in any way.

This is a passive truth. Yeah, the word abortion cannot be found in the bible, but there are places where God talked about a woman losing her child. This scripture is found in **Exodus 21: 22-24.**

"If men fight, and hurt a woman with child, so that she gives birth prematurely, yet no harm follows, he shall surely be punished accordingly as the woman's husband imposes on him; and he shall pay as the judges determine.

23 But if any harm follows, then you shall give life for life,

24 eye for eye, tooth for tooth, hand for hand, foot for foot..."

From this scripture, we can see God punishing a man for mistakenly taking out the child of a woman. How do you think God will address the woman if she takes out the child herself?

Note that the man didn't injure the woman, he only caused her to give birth prematurely, and God is commanding this great punishment on him; how much more when the woman takes the child out prematurely?

We have studied a lot of human theory in our time that has blinded our eyes to the truth in God's word. Indeed, these theories can be educational and blinding. There are a lot of theories that are enhanced which goes against the scripture.

The sperm of the man contains the seed of life, and when it mutates with the woman's egg, life is generated. That life is the growing child in the womb of the woman.

Ps 139:13-16

For You formed my inward parts;

You covered me in my mother's womb.

14 I will praise You, for I am fearfully and wonderfully made;

Marvelous are Your works,

And that my soul knows very well.

15 My frame was not hidden from You,

When I was made in secret,

And skillfully wrought in the lowest parts of the earth.

16 Your eyes saw my substance, being yet unformed.

And in Your book they all were written,

The days fashioned for me,

When as yet there were none of them.

Life doesn't begin when the child is fully made and given birth to, our life starts at the very point of conception, and God is so keen to take in all of these details. He knows the time life was created and that his seed is born. He sees through all the growth process and is very interested in what happens to the seed during development. You can see in verse 13, the writer explained that God covered him in his mother's womb. He mentioned that his days were already marked before God, so to God he was counted as a living being already.

There is a story of a young boy named Samuel Armas, at 21 weeks of gestation, he was operated on to correct his spina bifdia lesion at Vanderbilt University in 1999. He survived the operation, and today is a simmer. This further proves that the argument that the pregnancy contains just a fetus is not scientific or scriptural but a jumble from philosophy and emotions. If a baby of 21 weeks could be operated on, how dare we claim that it is just tissue in the womb?"

Another scripture that points out this truth is in **Jeremiah 1:5**

"I formed you in the womb I knew you;

Before you were born I sanctified you;

I ordained you a prophet to the nations."

From this scripture, we can see that God identified Jeremiah as a person, even when he was yet unborn. God formed him as a person and positioned him in his mother's womb.

This scripture is not what science can explain or validate. So, Jeremiah was existing from his mother's womb.

There are also other scriptures that amplify that an unborn child right from conception is a living being. We will be looking at some scriptures to highlight this point now.

Isa 49:1

"Listen, O coastlands, to Me,

And take heed, you peoples from afar!

The Lord has called Me from the womb;

From the matrix of My mother He has made mention of My name.

Gen 25:23-24

And the Lord said to her:

"Two nations are in your womb,

Two peoples shall be separated from your body;

One people shall be stronger than the other,

And the older shall serve the younger."

24 So when her days were fulfilled for her to give birth, indeed there were twins in her womb.

Judge 13:5

For behold, you shall conceive and bear a son. And no razor shall come upon his head, for the child shall be a Nazirite to God from the womb; and he shall begin to deliver Israel out of the hand of the Philistines."

These scriptures altogether show us that the unborn child, even at day one, is a living being, identified by God and commissioned with a purpose.

God said to Rachel that she has two nations in her womb. There is a mystery of the seed of a man that we need to understand. God blessed

Abraham and his seeds; who are the seeds of Abraham?

Of course, the many children that will come from his children's children. Many generations were blessed by Abraham, just because they are his seeds.

So, you were already existing in your parents' loins waiting for activation of life, which happens during sex.

Inside of you and I lie seeds of nations waiting for activation. When one of them is activated, it is no longer a seed but a fruit.

Ps 127:3

Behold, children are a heritage from the Lord,

The fruit of the womb is a reward

How then can we claim that it was only a fetus or tissue that was removed during abortion?

An entire seed that has been created, marked, and commissioned by God was actually what was eliminated from planet earth. Just like Jeremiah was ordained from the womb to be a prophet, so has God ordained every activated seed with an office and a glory. Eliminating that seed is called murder.

Having established that an unborn child is a human with life, we need also to establish that God is mindful of every life, and taking of life is murder before God.

Hence, according to scripture, termination of a fetus by abortion is murder!

Chapter Two

The weight/cost of abortion

From time to time, we keep raising arguments over this matter. Several debates have been held to oppose or support the idea of abortion. However, there never seems to be a pronounced answer after all. The decision is always left for the government to make.

Nonetheless, the average person keeps asking if indeed abortion is wrong or not? We keep asking these questions in our local groups, churches and on the streets. There is a salient search for validation and fear of judgment or consequence.

The proponents of abortion have been of the stance for many years that abortion isn't wrong. They believe it is some bunch of religious jargon that makes people feel uncomfortable with it. Their chant is hinged around the fact that it is a woman's right to decide what she wants to do to her body. They give the following reasons why it is not wrong to have an abortion.

1. **Women should have control over their body**: Just as we have highlighted, this is a major reason this movement is thriving and advancing by the day. People love to hear something logical and sentimental at the same time. Anything that is validated upon such

a premise will always be championed and supported by majority and politicized. The former American president, Bill Clinton, went ahead to support abortions saying all should be safe, legal, and rare. This means, it shouldn't be done every time, and the method of abortion must be safe, done through the right process and at the right place. They also believe that you don't owe anyone an explanation for what is going on.

2. **They believe that abortion is just the removal of tissue and nothing more**: we have discussed this in the previous chapter. This is fact-less by scripture and science. We have established that from conception, a seed of life is planted

and begins to grow as a person. This gospel is something they disagree with; they believe that pregnancy is a possibility, not actually a person.

3. **Abortion is morally good**: 'if you are not ready for it, get rid of it', they say. It is also justified as a health care system; a way of keeping the body healthy and sound. A popular western official once said in an international interview that, all women are pro-life activists, but there are circumstances whereby that is the only means of handling it. She says it should not be cancelled because some people are not comfortable with it as it isn't wrong in itself. This we know not to be true also. There is nothing moral about

abortion. It is just a self-preservation technique from responsibility. Abortion is the route to avoiding responsibility or pain from a pregnancy conceived in error; they believe the baby is not subject to feelings so it is wrong to suffer or punish the mother to take responsibility when the process isn't hurting the baby.

4. **The scripture is silent concerning it, there's no mention of abortion anywhere in the scriptures:** We've dealt on this already in chapter one. There's nothing the Bible is silent about. We need to understand that. The Bible is our manual of life.

All manuals guide the use of its product. So, there's no issue that a product will have that can't be addressed by the manual. There is none whatsoever! The product manufacturer actually knows the peak of pressure the product can take, what it should be used to do, how to prevent it from breaking down, maintenance tips, and what to do when it breaks down.

Same with God. As our creator, he has created a manual for life, so we have the Bible as a manual, given to us by God, so we have to report to the book when in need of life for strength and guidance.

But abortion is not the problem in itself. There's a heart state that is not at peace with it.

Again, there's something in you that is against evil. Yes, I know you have heard that man is full of sin, that he was born and bred in the evil nature called sin, so he doesn't have any good in him. That's not true!

God breathed his breath upon man during creation, there's a deposit of God in every man, that deposit is called CONSCIENCE. After man ate the forbidden fruit, his eyes were open to good and evil.

The identifying factor was not his physical eyes but his conscience. When we begin to do evil, there's an unsettlement in our hearts, and we start to check. Is this actually right and wrong?

Conscience is that thing that makes you begin to check if actually Abortion is right. Asides the so many views people have given in support for or against abortion, there is a silent feeling of discomfort you have with the whole idea.

Deep down in your conscience, you feel this is wrong. You can't explain it but you're not just so comfortable with it. What about the pain and emotional loss? There is just this thing that makes you feel not to at peace with the decision. In as much as some persons walk in and out of the abortion theater acting like they have just done nothing but treated a disease, 80% of women that have had abortion say that they are never comfortable with the process or the decision, but many times they are stuck with no other option, and abortion seems to be the only escape route they know out of their mistake. It is an unpleasable thing no woman wishes to do until she finds herself with a mistake in her womb.

They go ahead to silence the voice in their head and argue reasons why abortion isn't bad. They begin to bring up arguments, theories, and logic to prove against what the scripture is saying and what their conscience is telling them. These folks do this over and over until their conscience is dead. They become dead spiritually and cease to feel the burden that something is wrong or not. They have been handed over to their logic and feeling.

This set of people then seek to Lord their logical lifestyle over others and cause everyone to begin to defy the voice of their conscience that speaks truth, which is the voice of God.

This brings us down to what this whole battle is about. It is the battle against the truth as I said, and the spirit of the Antichrist that has risen to validate things that are against the word of God.

Abortion is just one of those things. However, those that are true in spirit with God can never align to such a plan. Those that still have their conscience alive can never stand fully stand and support this movement.

Although they have been attacked time after time by feminists worldwide, the pro-life are bent on exposing the reality of abortion and its consequences to the world. They are ready to go to any extent to campaign against this criminal activity, as they term it.

Below are some of the reasons why the pro-life fight against abortion.

1. They believe that the life of a woman is equal to that of the baby she is carrying: the pro-life campaign that every fetus baby is deserving of

life. They are against prioritizing women over their babies. Their first and top reason for fighting is the fact that abortion kills a person. They believe the abortion patients should be punished for murder. This is the one unified belief pro-life activists have worldwide. Other things are championed by small pro-life groups and sometimes contradict themselves. However, every pro-life anywhere in the world opposes abortion because they believe it is against human life.

2.	They assert that no one really wants an abortion. If there were any other option to solve their problems, women would gladly go for it, but abortion seems to be the only way of getting rid of an unwanted pregnancy.

3. Reduction in population: The pro-life activists who share in this belief, even as unreligious persons, point out that abortion has killed three times the number of children who died in wars and disease breakouts. Can you imagine such a figure! Abortion influences the national population uncontrollably. This downsize is not controllable by even the government. It is a national waste of potential human resources.

4. It is selfish.: The pro-life believes that in no way is the woman's life highly valuable than that of the child. The child is as much of a human as

is the child and has a right to life. Killing the child is depriving that child of living. Doing it because of some personal reasons is as wicked as directly murder. The life of an unborn child is a costly expense to sacrifice because of unpreparedness or whatever excuses.

5. Abortion always leads to grief: The proponents of abortion try to argue this truth but it is a fact that they can't eliminate no matter how hard they try to silence the truth. Unlike the proponents feel that it is inconsequential and just a sincere removal of a mistaken pregnancy, pro-life clearly states that abortion

could lead to deep grief and depression.

Well, there might be a pregnancy by mistake but there's no mistaken child. Every seed that entered into this world was ordained to do so from the day of conception. He was given a mandate.

No one can tell how exactly a child is formed in the womb of a woman, not even science. How did the ears come out? The hands and everything? How did the sperm fuse with egg and gain so much relevance. It is obviously a miracle; the work of a supernatural being the world is beginning to turn away from. One out of millions of sperm successfully hit it and became a child. Isn't that a miracle?

Terminating that pregnancy is wasting that miracle!!

In chapter one, we have established that abortion is murder, and according to scripture, murder is wrong and a sin against God. Having established that, we know that everything wrong has its consequences.

The fear of facing these unknown consequences causes many to keep asking, 'is abortion wrong?' despite all the debates that have been held for and against it.

Indirectly, they ask, is there a consequence I need to be afraid of if I go ahead to have an abortion?

Well, the pro-life activists are of the opinion that abortion is highly consequential to the state, not just one person.

Let us see what the bible has to say about this.

Is There Any Consequence Of Abortion Stated In The Scripture?

1. Eternal death: The gospel states that every sin is punishable by God. God is a holy God and cannot behold iniquity.

However, it is not more serious than other sins. There is no big sin or small sin. Abortion is as punishable as lying and stealing. Although many religious persons try to make it look like the greatest sin of all time only to discourage people from engaging in it. The gospel truth is that; every single sin is equal before the sight of God.

Gal 5:19-23

19 The acts of the sinful nature are obvious: sexual immorality, impurity and debauchery; 20 idolatry and witchcraft; hatred, discord, jealousy, fits of rage, selfish ambition, dissensions, factions 21 and envy; drunkenness, orgies, and the like. I warn you, as I did before, that those who live like this will not inherit the kingdom of God.

(New International Version, NIV)

According to this scripture, those who engage in sexual immorality will never inherit the kingdom of God. New King James Version also includes the sin of murder, which is also abortion. There are two destinations after life; heaven (eternal life) and hell (eternal death).

Hence, if scripture says a person will not inherit God's kingdom, it means that they will be headed into hell for eternal death and destruction.

Rev 20:15

And anyone not found written in the Book of Life was cast into the lake of fire.

The book of life contains the names of those who have lived right and will spend their eternity in heaven. Anyone whose name is not in this book is doomed for hell. Therefore, the abortionist and all other sinners who don't repent are in danger of hell. The very first consequence of abortion, according to scripture, is eternal death.

2. Spiritual death; this is the death of the conscience. Once a person gives himself to sin, he kills his conscience. If you study persons that committed several abortions, you'll notice that many of them are hardened. Once a person commits his soul to sin, his soul is disconnected

from God. This is not just for the abortionist but every soul that sins. Anyone that makes a habit of sin has separated himself from the covering of God.

1 Tim 4:2

2 Speaking lies in hypocrisy; having their conscience seared with a hot iron;

This is the position of anyone that consistently give into sin, all manner of sin, not just abortion, they always have this terrible hardness of heart.

Titus 1:15

15 Unto the pure all things are pure: but unto them that are

defiled and unbelieving is nothing pure; but even their mind and conscience is defiled.

Their conscience is defiled, and their mind is defiled. They are spiritually dead and cannot connect with God. There is always this wall of defilement between them and God, breaching their access to God.

3. Health complications: In countries like Africa where Abortion is not legal, it is clandestinely performed by unskilled practitioners using hazardous devices in a dirty environment. This could lead to complications in the next pregnancy,

stillbirth of the baby, rupturing of the womb, and sepsis.

Typical complications are bleeding, remains of the pregnancy, infections like PID pelvic inflammatory disease. Asides from these, there could also be silent problems that could come up and be very disturbing. One of such cases is a lady who after having an abortion started to have excruciating cramps. Though there are professional and safer abortion procedures; it still can't be fully trusted.

4. Waste of divine destinies: This is a heavy cost of abortion that is highlighted also in the Alabama abortion ban which happens to be one of the strictest ban there is. God

said that all souls are precious to him; taking away one soul is very costly.

Just imagine the futures that go to waste as a result of abortion. The number of children that are killed every year. What if the next Abraham Lincoln is one of those children or Kathryn Kulman. Divine destinies that God has mandated to transform their world, the Jeremiahs that are being deprived of life by selfish reasons. Abortion robs the world of divine destinies that God could use to cause transformation here on earth.

4. Trauma: the trauma from post abortions is one thing that affects many women that have had abortion especially after health complications.

A murderer and an abortionist will be tormented by their conscience and guilt for a long time.

A murderer haunted by guilt is doomed — there's no helping him.

Prov 28:17

Some abortionists claim to be hunted by the spirit of their baby. For some, there's just this restlessness and guilt. You might wonder if these things really happen why do people still do abortions. This subject matter will be well discussed in the last chapter of this book; ensure you patiently read through and allow your spirit to be blessed.

Chapter Three

The Alternative to Abortion

Except to save a woman's life, abortion still remains illegal in many places. The few countries where abortion are legalized are: U. S, Tunisia, New Zealand, Denmark, Belgium, Austria, France, Sweden, Netherlands, and Italy. If you don't stay in any of these places, you would have to find an alternative to abortion.

Well, anyone could always still have their abortion in a low life health center (I mean, those guys are existent everywhere), but having read through the last two chapters, I believe the thought of abortion should be least considered now.

An unexpected pregnancy can be tough to deal with. You are confused, perplexed and nervous. You are pregnant with a baby you don't want to have; you are looking for viable options that could help you lift the burden on your shoulders.

For all the burdens in the world, abortion is no option, and there's no virtually way to go about it than to face it. The other alternatives you have comes after birth. Yes! You would have to carry the baby till its time and deliver.

There are series of options open to you and very viable. However, none of them will help you terminate the baby. You would have to carry the baby till delivery before any of these options can work for you. They will help you handle the stress and responsibilities that come afterward. You have to face it and bear the consequence of your mistake if you think it is one. Having the baby is owning that you are wrong and wise enough to take responsibility for your actions.

Below are three alternatives for abortion and are in no way contradictory with scriptures.

1. Adoption: this is the legal transfer of custody and parenting rights of your child to another family. It is of two

types; open and closed, and two forms; agency and direct placement.

a. Open adoption: Here, the family agrees to grant you access to the child through calls, texts, and visits once in a while. They also give you updates, invite you for occasional dinner and encourage the child to reach out to you once he/she is at a particular age. The medium and measure of access will be discussed during the signing of the papers.

b. Closed adoption: if you choose a closed adoption,

you will be signing your goodbye to your child, as this form of adoption withholds all forms of access. Your child won't know you are his parent, except his adoptive family decides to inform him. If they do so, he will be allowed to see the adoption papers by age 18.

c. Agency: giving your child away through an agency who will connect you to an adoptive parent. there are so many adoption agencies in town. You need to be sure you are dealing with the right one. Make sure to go for the one that makes you feel more relaxed and provide honest answers to your question, the agency that supports you and helps you access medical care. Finally, it must be licensed.

d. Direct placement: this is you selecting an adoptive family yourself on your own grounds. There is a need for the help of an adoption attorney for a direct placement. The legal fees should be covered by the adoptive family, after which the attorney helps you decide between an open and closed adoption using the details you provided.

The process of adoption is never easy. Talk about parting away with a child you carried in your womb for nine months and giving him/her out. That is not easy. However, it saves you from committing the sin and crime of murder.

2. Legal guardianship: Just like adoption, this involves the giving away of your child plus parenting rights to a different family, which is most times a close relative, church member

or family friend. However, it is for a short time and requires some level of financial commitment from you. To initiate this process, you will need to hire an attorney to help you with official documents for you and your child's guardian. The time frame of guardianship and agreed commitment fee will be fixed before the process is properly initiated.
3. Parenting: You never considered parenting before now, but it is still a viable option you could consider. Motherhood is as rewarding as it is stressful. If you are

considering this option, there are two forms of parenting:

a. Co-parenting: this involves you and the child's parent jointly raising the child together. This is an excellent and workable option if your partner supports the idea, and is in good terms with you. If the relationship was abusive or your partner isn't interested in accepting the fatherhood role, you should consider single parenting.

b. Single parenting: Many people dread this more than anything; it is the main reason why many opt for adoption. Single parenthood is not a death sentence. Some people chose this option, and today they have no regrets whatsoever. Indeed, single parenting can be challenging, but it is much easier when there is support. Endeavor to use the support of family and friends when you feel you need it. Never try to punish yourself and take in the whole pressure. Use some help!

Now, we will be revisiting our list of reasons why people commit abortion and prescribe the best alternatives to each reason.

Bad timing, not prepared. This is one of the most popular reasons people give for aborting their baby. Associated reasons could be that the pregnancy interferes with their educational or career goals. We have many career women who are presently have had to eliminate many mistake pregnancies.

Adoption and legal guardianship are two options to be considered. If you would want to keep the baby years later, but you are not prepared because of school or your career, guardianship is a viable option to consider. Guardianship could also work for you as a married career woman. If your spouse has no problems with it, you could give the child to a close relative for some years, until you are ready.

Not emotionally and mentally prepared: This set of people give the excuse that they are not ready for motherhood's responsibility.

Nobody knows how prepared they are for motherhood until they give it a try. Motherhood is a course you learn on the go, so if this is your only excuse, don't be afraid to try parenting. Your worry about meeting the responsibility of motherhood is a sign that you'll make a good mother. There are training organizations that could also train you on parenting and grant you financial support.

Rape case: 98% of pregnant rape victims abort their baby because of the pain and trauma.

Most pregnant rape victims are known to hate their child strongly. The pain and trauma of having a child for someone you have come to hate and probably do not know can be overwhelming. If you are in such shoes, adoption is an option you should consider. However, you could still keep the child if you are not traumatized by its existent.

Partner-related reasons: when a lady gets pregnant in an abusive or new relationship, she hurriedly gets rid of the baby. She is scared of having a child for someone who might turn them and the baby down and eventually walk away, leaving her a single mother.

This has been addressed above. Single motherhood is not a death sentence; you can give it a try.

None of these alternatives are easy. Having to give away a baby you carried for nine months and choosing to be a parent when you were never prepared is a big deal. However, there are organizations to help you. Whatever alternative you decide, you don't need to do it alone. *Planned parenthood* is one organization that is committed to helping young pregnant women, they also render counseling services if you ever have a problem making the decision.

Maintaining purity

You shouldn't bring a child into the world if you're not ready for the responsibility. However, no one talks about the process. We all condemn or decide on the product (the baby), but fail to talk about the process that led to the pregnancy. No one just gets pregnant, sex leads to pregnancy and although there are a lot of contraceptives that people use today, none of them is 100% guaranteed. Pregnancy is still possible even if the couple doesn't will it.

What you call a mistake is a destined child, who was planned to come later but by your carelessness or worldliness you brought it to being now. I'm not saying that everything that happens is God's plan, and we just let it, NO!

God is sovereign; his ways are not our ways. His words are final, yes but when it comes to decision making, he has entrusted that into our hands.

Right after creation, he said choose ye this day death and life. So we have the choice to make. Don't listen to anyone who tells you God will and orders everything till the tiniest detail isn't telling all of the truth. We still have our way of influencing his will.

He has written his heart and will in the Scriptures to guide us to live how we wants. Hence, if everyone lives according to the scripture, we're sure to have the world running according to his will, but we're subject to our will. God has established the ordinance of the world and given us resources to do the right things, but because of our stubbornness, we have chosen otherwise, and this is why our world is how it is today.

God's word says to run away from youthful lust and immorality, adultery, and fornication. If indeed we run away from these things, there'll be no pregnancy to abort. The whole worry of what to do will be unnecessary.

If you are not married, avoid sex! I think there's no better time than at this point to announce this to us.

Scripture regarded sex as honorable between couples alone. So even if you're married, you're licensed to have sex only with your spouse and no other person.

Staying sexually pure will save you from the hassle of trying to find an alternative for abortion, and it is very possible to stay pure.

In Titus 2:11-12, the scriptures says,

11 "For the grace of God that brings salvation has appeared unto all men

12 Teaching us that denying ungodliness and worldliness, we should live soberly, righteously, and godly in this present world."

The grace of God teaches and enables us to live right, and he said this grace has appeared unto ALL men. That means you and I have undeniable access to this grace. You have the grace to be sexually pure and say no to premarital sex.

However, if you have made the mistake, there is also grace for you to make the right choice and live right henceforth.

Chapter Four

What If I've Already Committed Abortion?

The Alabama abortion's ban proposes that abortionists be punished for murder, though it hasn't been made law. It is evident that people view abortionists as criminals that are worthy of punishment. This law is being practiced in some states as of present.

It is also no news that abortionists are been stigmatized worldwide. It is rare to see someone rise up to receive recognition as an abortionist, the stigma is real. Before the eyes of people, you are a condemned criminal and deserves to be punished. However, God doesn't look at you from that perspective.

Now you know that what you did was wrong; a sin against God and man. It is one thing to know and another to realize that and take the right decision towards that direction.

God said something very intriguing in **Isaiah 1:18**

"Come now, and let us reason together,"

Says the Lord,

"Though your sins are like scarlet,

They shall be as white as snow;

Though they are red like crimson,

They shall be as wool."

Did you see that? God says he will wipe away every one of your sins even though they be as dark as scarlet. Do you know what is scarlet? Bright red color! Even though your sins are bloody and dark, he will wipe all of them away, and that is the very end of every sin you have ever committed except nothing.

Even the sins of murder, abortion, and immorality will be forgiven. Every sin will be gone and you will be white as snow. Do you believe that?

Yes! That is the word of God and his word doesn't lie. Never!

But before he called you pure, did you see the first sentence? He said, 'come let us reason together.' God is calling you for a heart to heart. He wants to change you, and you know the first thing? He says, Come!

When we fall into sin, especially ones as powerful as this, what we do many times is to run from God, instead of running to God! the devil comes in and uses that opportunity to keep us farther. He savages you with guilt on all sides and then you settle to believe that God can never forgive you. You become so overladen with guilt and decide to turn to the world for succor. But you know what, there is no succor there. The only cleansing power is in the blood of Jesus. So he said, though your sin be dark, red, terrible, he is able and very willing to take it from you.

He went on further to say in **Matt 11:28,**

Come unto me, all ye that labour and are heavy ladened.

The devil may have filled you with guilt, making you feel unacceptable to God.

I come to tell you that he is a liar and the father of all liars. Because he won't want you to be comfortable with your walk with God, he doesn't want you anywhere near peace, love and joy. He keeps pulling you away and imprisons you with guilt.

It is time for you to answer that call and break away from the yoke of the devil. Yes, you have had several abortions, Jesus says, I don't condemn you. Come let me wash you clean again.

In Luke 5, when the Pharisees were rebuking Jesus for eating with the sinners, he asked a very sensitive question,

"To whom do the physician come, to the sick or to the whole?"

Why did Jesus come, why was his blood shed, if not to give you a new sheet and make you whole?

He said in **John 3: 16,** *"**for God so loved the world that he gave us***

his only begotten son. Whoever believes in him will not perish but have an everlasting life."

This popular scripture we've repeated all of our days in church has the answer in it. GOD DOESN'T CONDEMN YOU, DON'T LET THE DEVIL CONDEMN YOU. Don't allow the condemnation from people make you condemn yourself!

Yes, God is not happy about what you did, but he will rather have you with him than far from him, because he loves you. He knows we are weak in the flesh and cannot do some things that is why he has sent his son to us. He didn't die for nothing, his blood was to cleanse us and cover for our weaknesses. The blood of Jesus is more than sufficient for you.

Hence, the first thing you can do is GO TO GOD.

Ask him to come into your life. Ask him to make you clean and watch the transformation that will unfold. So, as I have established, the first step is talking to and with God.

Next, join a bible believing church where you can grow in the world and faith.

Such an atmosphere will help you grow in the faith and increase your love for God. When your love for God is increased, the more passion you have to serve God, the bigger the testimony. Just as Heb 10:22

highlights, now that you have given your life to God, you need to draw nearer. Joining a church will teach you how you can draw closer to God.

Heb 10:22

22 Let us draw near with a true heart in full assurance of faith, having our hearts sprinkled from an evil conscience, and our bodies washed with pure water.

Also, endeavor to go for counselling and join a support group. You might need to visit the counsellor and join a support group. After you have talked to God, you might still feel the need to speak to someone for empathy sake. Do not fail to see the counsellor or join a support group if there is anyone around you. In some countries, there are local district groups you could join if you desire to. Joining a church assembly will also help you take one step further on number one decision; it will help provide you moral support.

Finally, you need to restitute.

You might be wondering what restitution has to do with abortion. Well, this doesn't apply to all situations. If you had it at the back of your parents, spouse, or pastor, you might have to confess it to them. By that, you are restituting. But don't do any of this if you haven't done step one and two. They will help to prepare your heart to do such.

Plus there is this peace that comes with confession, it exposes you to a form of prosperity.

Jesus says, "**he that covereth his sin will not prosper.**" You need to unveil and talk to those that need to know about it.

Once you have done all of this, try to abstain totally from sex. Now you are pure, do not defile yourself any longer. Abstain from any form of sexual immorality.

Ps 32:1-2

Blessed is he whose transgression is forgiven, whose sin is covered.

2 Blessed is the man unto whom the Lord imputeth not iniquity, and in whose spirit there is no guile.

Prayer for healing

Dear Lord, I had an abortion thinking it was my best option, but the grief and guilt I have felt ever since I took that decision has haunted me, and I feel so ashamed of myself and pierced with guilt. My heart is so heavy and I find that I am not able to think about anything else and I realize each day that it is against Your Principles Lord, that I have sinned and done this great wrong to my child and myself.

Father Lord, I feel broken inside and need Your comfort and healing. You have promised to repair the brokenhearted and to set those that with guilt and shame free, and Lord, you have promised forgiveness and restoration to all who humbly come to Your throne of mercy and grace to confess their transgression. My hope is in You, for You alone can restore the joy of my salvation.

Thank You, for You are a forgiving God, whose mercies renew every morning and so I hand this over to You today, and ask for the healing and restoration that only You can give, and the grace to forget my mistake and move on, following your divine principles. I ask this through Christ our Lord, Amen.

Chapter Five

Dealing with post abortion trauma

This is one problem most abortionists face and are silent about. You hear people try to shrug off anti-abortion talks. They try to nullify the possibility of a complication, depression or emotional trauma.

They go on speaking about people they know that have had abortion countless times and still happens to be living their life to the fullness. Well, it might be true that with the aid of drugs, post-abortion complications can be avoided. However, no drug can take care of the trauma.

Most abortionists hide their trauma, so no one can suspect anything. They use pretense smiles and acts to make people believe they are fine while they are hide a deep rooted pain.

Statistics has it that about 80% of abortionists face traumas.

That is a very alarming percentage. Though most people get over the traumatic feeling after a while, many more are caged by it throughout their lifetime.

Before we move further, let's put a peg here and define trauma.

Trauma is defined as a severe emotional shock and pain caused by an extremely upsetting experience. It is characterized by pain, loss and emotional emptiness; it is as though a part of you was ripped out, which is true in some way. That child was a part of you, and removing the child will surely leave a heavy vacuum. Standing up from that theatre bed or watching that baby flush down the toilet, you feel empty and heavy all of a sudden. Like you just lost a significant part of you and for a long time, that feeling stays, leaving you emotionally stressed and confused. Such feelings rid you of productivity and could translate into physical ailments like hypertension.

In worse cases, there are feelings of guilt, anger, shame, lack of self-confidence, and thoughts of suicide.

There is a case of a girl who had committed several abortions, she broke down in tears when interviewed and confessed that she was continually plagued by suicidal thoughts after that incidence.

Another woman said that the cries of babies get her restless and reminds her of her aborted child. Many women claim to hear or see their baby's voice calling out to them. Others seem to be drowned in different forms of guilt and grief.

A popular story is told of a young lady of 16 who had her first abortion, she had no complications, but it was only a matter of time before she fell depressed. She felt she didn't deserve to live because she had killed her baby. The thoughts were driving her nuts, alongside her depression. She was about committing suicide when she found a counselling center that helped relieve her from pain. Around that time, she started attending church with her boyfriend and one day, heard a message from a woman talking about abortion and its effect on women. The story blew her away and she realized fully what she had done and repented before God.

She reached out to join the ministry to reach out to the women, but they counselled her to pass through a healing class first. From her story and that of other survivors, we can draw a few tips.

1. Forgiveness: After the deed has been done, you feel you shouldn't have done it, and you are angry with yourself. This anger can lead to depression if not well handled. This is why forgiveness is very important. It is the first process any counselling section will take you through. Forgive yourself! God has forgiven you, so what is holding back from forgiving yourself? Let the guilt go!

2. Join a support group: you could join a support group that's nearest to you. It can be very therapeutic. One beautiful thing about joining a support group, it allows you to be in a place of like minds. Here the stories of others and share yours without feeling judged or condemned. It isn't

just therapeutic but educative. Suggestion on books to read, movies to read and things to do at depressive moments are necessary information you cannot find anywhere else. A support group can help you get over quickly.

3. Offer to volunteer for pro-life campaigns: From one of the survivor's stories we read, you can see that her motivation to volunteer helped her find freedom. When you set out to educate young persons and rally against abortion, you are liberating yourself and at the same time saving lives. Talk about it everywhere; you could mobilize your church members and friends. What is important is that you are doing

something to fight abortion. It has a way of perfecting and accelerating your healing process. The joy and satisfaction that comes from the knowledge that you are saving a life is helping so much that when depressive thoughts try to grip you down, you can gain strength in the knowledge that you have brought help to someone that was about to make the same mistake you made in the past.

Conclusion

Abortion is not just a debate topic but a missile from the devil into the world, especially in this generation. He knows lawlessness is against the ways of God and very displeasing to him, so he tries to trap us into it by giving us reasons upon reasons why wrong is right. And many times, we almost succumb to his wiles and deception in many forms

He makes the truth appear as false and false as truth; this way, he susceptibly leads people to follow his practices and believe in his doctrine. He sets a trap on the beautiful sands of gold that only the wise can avoid and the surest way to resist his traps is to avoiding trailing on those sands.

In this brief illustration, the sands of gold represent premarital sex, and the trap is abortion. These are two sins linked together and championed by the anti-Christ, which is the devil. He has watered down strategically, every form of conviction that is held over these things.

He tries to make them appear normal to us. Anytime you see men trying to feel normal about what is universally wrong and having thick arguments on whether to go against or in support of it, that is the spirit of the antichrist at work. The bible says the spirit of the anti-Christ will be dominating in the last days.

1 John 2:18

Little children, it is the last time: and as ye have heard that antichrist shall come, even now are there many antichrists; whereby we know that it is the last time.

We are in the end times, the last days before the end of the world, and the devil knows his time would soon be up on earth so he is trying everything possible to trap people through whatsoever means. It is not only the issue of fornication and abortion he has watered, the devil has tried to reduce and water down every standard of God to stray many away from the truth therefore leading them to eternal damnation. He has gone as far as making people believe that God is not in existence, giving them theories and cogent reasons why they shouldn't believe in God. Today in most of Europe the percentage of people who don't believe in God or any form of religion has multiplied.

He makes the world see God and his ways as bondage and sin a liberation. The bible warned and gave us signs of the anti-Christ.

1 John 4:2-3

By this you know the Spirit of God: Every spirit that confesses that Jesus Christ has come in the flesh is of God, and every spirit that does not confess that

Jesus Christ has come in the flesh is not of God. And this is the spirit of the Antichrist, which you have heard was coming, and is now already in the world.

You will agree with me that many people who applaud abortion and other evils trending today don't believe in God; They also disagree with any statement that Jesus is the Son of God and that he came into the world to die for mankind. Logic, science and philosophy have taken over the minds of many. This is an operation of the anti-Christ.

Another thing to know is that abortion is also a trap by the anti-Christ to steal divine destinies before their time. It is not a new strategy, the devil used this strategy in the time of Moses and Jesus. Sincerely, I have wondered what those children that were aborted would have turned out to be if they were given a chance to live. Abortion is a menacing trap. It is worse in our time because he is using us against us. That is causing us to sin against God while we take away precious destinies. It is high time we stand up angrily and change the game.

I want you to know one last thing that Jesus thinks about abortion;

'it is a sin and a sharp system of the antichrist."

The antichrist knows that many young persons want to be free, they want to enjoy life to the fullest and have all manner of fun. Hence he has introduced lawlessness to the system. Many that are no wise have grabbed this as an opportunity for them to live their life carelessly.

1 John 3:4-9

Whoever commits sin also commits lawlessness, and sin is lawlessness. 5 And you know that He was manifested to take away our sins, and in Him there is no sin. 6 Whoever abides in Him does not sin. Whoever sins has neither seen Him nor known Him.

7 Little children, let no one deceive you. He who practices righteousness is righteous, just as He is righteous. 8 He who sins is of the devil, for the devil has sinned from the beginning. For this purpose, the Son of God was manifested, that He might destroy the works of the devil.

Do not accept any form of lawlessness! It is a trap from the devil. Jesus came to destroy the work of the devil. What is that work? Normalizing lawlessness! God is love, and he is a God of lawful principles.

What this means is that God has a set of regulations, and yet he helps us carry this out with love.

Jesus is saying, come to me all ye that are burdened. Come to me all ye that are labored.

You know the truth. Live the truth. Yes, you might be the only one acting the right way, but one light has to shine and show others the way.

You can be nobly holy!

You can live the truth!

You can be sexually pure!

You can have an abortion free life!

Yes! I know you can, and I am rooting for you, deeply.

Prayer

Eternal God, We praise You for the Fatherly care which You extend to all creation, especially to us, made in Your image and likeness.

Father, extend Your hand of protection to those babies threatened by abortion and save them from its destructive power. Give Your strength to all mothers and fathers that they may never give in to the fears tempting them to facilitate abortions.

I am ready to do my part in ending abortion. Today I commit myself Never to be silent, never to be passive, Or forgetful of the unborn child.

I commit myself to be active in the pro-life movement, never to stop defending human life until all my sisters and brothers are protected!

Bless our families and bless our land, that we may have the joy of welcoming and nurturing the life of which You are the source through Christ our Lord. Amen!

www.ingramcontent.com/pod-product-compliance
Lightning Source LLC
Chambersburg PA
CBHW070424220526
45466CB00004B/1530